GOOD POSTURE, HEALTHY LIFE:

TIPS ON HOW TO LEAD A PAINLESS LIFE

BY

B. O EMMA

TABLE OF CONTENTS

INTRODUCTION

Activities and tips to assist with reducing muscle strain brought about by unfortunate sitting and standing propensities.

Physiotherapist Scratch Sinfield depicts 8 normal stance slip-ups and how to address them with strength and extending works out. Assuming you have back torment, further developing your stance is probably not going to address the main driver of your aggravation, however, it might assist with mitigating muscle pressure.

"Revising your stance might feel off-kilter at first because your body has become so used to sitting and remaining with a specific goal in mind," says Sinfield.

"Yet, with a touch of training, the great stance will turn out to be natural and be 1 stage to aiding your back in the long haul."

The nuts and bolts of Stance

The act is how you hold your body while standing, sitting, or performing errands like lifting, twisting, pulling, or coming to. Assuming that your stance is great, the bones of the spine — the vertebrae — are accurately adjusted.

Normal stance mix-ups and fixes

1. Collapsing in a seat

Collapsing doesn't necessarily in every case cause uneasiness, however, over the long haul, this position can overburden previously sharpened muscles and delicate tissues. This strain might increment pressure in the muscles, which may thusly cause torment.

Start sitting accurately. It may not feel good at first because your muscles have not been adapted to help you in the right position. Activities to reinforce your center and butt cheek muscles, and back expansions will assist with revising a slumping stance.

2. Staying your base out

f your base will in general stand out or you have an articulated bend in your lower back, you might have hyperlordosis. This is a misrepresented internal bend of the lower back that makes a "Donald Duck" pose.

Center and butt cheek reinforcing work out, hip flexor and thigh stretch, and putting forth a cognizant attempt to address your standing stance are prescribed to assist with rectifying a standing out the base. Wearing high heels, unnecessary load around the stomach, and pregnancy can all add to a "Donald Duck" act.

To assist with revising your standing stance, envision a string joined to the highest point of your head pulling you upwards. The thought is to keep your body in amazing arrangement, keeping up with the spine's normal arch, with your neck straight and shoulders lined up with the hips: keep your shoulders back and loosened up pull in your mid-region keep your feet about hip distance separated balance your weight equally on the two feet make an effort not to shift your head forward, in reverse or sideways keep your legs straight, yet knees loose

3. Remaining with a level back

A level back implies your pelvis is wrapped up and your lower back is straight rather than normally bent, making you stoop forward. Individuals with a level back frequently track down it troublesome representing extensive stretches

This stance is frequently brought about by muscle uneven characters, which urge you to embrace such a position. Spending extensive stretches plunking down can likewise add to a level back. A level back likewise will in general make you lean your neck and head advance, which can cause neck and upper back strain. Activities to fortify your center, posterior, neck, and back shoulder muscles, and back expansions, are prescribed to assist with revising a level back.

4. Resting on 1 leg

Resting more on 1 leg while standing can feel good, particularly on the off chance that you have been representing for some time. Be that as it may, rather than utilizing your bottom and center muscles to keep you upstanding, you put exorbitant tension on 1 side of your lower back and hip.

After some time, you might foster muscle irregular characteristics around the pelvis region, which can cause solid strain in the lower back and rear end. Different reasons for lopsided hips remember conveying weighty knapsacks for 1 shoulder, and guardians conveying little children on 1 hip. To work on this stance, attempt to start remaining with your weight equitably dispersed on the two legs.

5. Slouched back and 'text neck'

Slouching over your console is normally a sign that you have a tight chest and a feeble upper back. Over the long run, this sort of stance can add to you fostering an adjusted upper back, which can cause shoulder and upper back solidness.

While slouching over a PC, your head might more often than not incline forward, which can prompt an unfortunate stance. Utilizing a versatile can lead to comparative issues named "text neck". Upper back, neck, and back shoulder fortifying activities, chest stretches, and neck act drills are prescribed to assist with remedying a slouched back.

6. Jabbing your jawline

The jabbing jawline stance can be brought about by sitting too low, a screen set excessively high, a slouched back, or a mix of each of the 3.

Revising a jabbing jawline includes working on your sitting propensities and activities to address your stance.

Instructions to address a jabbing jaw:

Tenderly extend your neck upwards as you wrap up your jawline cut your shoulder bones down and back towards your spine pull in your lower belly muscles to keep a characteristic bend in your lower back and change your seating.

7. Adjusted shoulders

A method for telling on the off chance that you have adjusted your shoulders is to remain before a mirror and allowed your arms to hang normally by your sides. Assuming that your knuckles look ahead, it might demonstrate that you have a tight chest and a feeble upper back, given the presence of adjusted shoulders.

Adjusted shoulders are normally brought about by unfortunate stance propensities, muscle irregular characteristics, and zeroing in a lot on specific activities, for example, a lot of spotlight on chest strength while ignoring the upper back.

8. Supporting your telephone.

Holding your telephone handset between your ear and shoulder overwhelms the muscles of the neck, upper back, and shoulders. The neck and shoulders are not intended to stand firm on this footing for any timeframe.

Over the long run, this stance can overburden the muscles and other delicate tissues, and lead to muscle irregular characteristics between the left and right sides of your neck.

Attempt to start holding the telephone with your hand, or utilizing a sans hands gadget.

Practices for neck firmness and torment:

The neck extends - delicately bring down your left ear towards your left shoulder; hold for 10 to 15 full breaths, then recurrent on the contrary side

Neck revolutions - gradually turn your jaw towards 1 shoulder; hold for 10 to 15 full breaths, then recurrent on the contrary side

4 methods for transforming a great stance into less back torment

You can work on your stance — and head off back torment — by rehearsing a few symbolism and a couple of simple activities.

Symbolism: Consider a straight line going through your body from roof to floor (your ears, shoulders, hips, knees, and lower legs ought to be even and line up upward). Presently envision that a solid string joined to the highest point of your head is pulling you vertical, making you taller. Attempt to hold your pelvis level — don't permit the lower back to influence — and fight the temptation to remain stealthily. All things considered, consider extending your head toward the roof, expanding the space between your rib enclosure and pelvis. Envision yourself as a ballet dancer or ice skater instead of a trooper at consideration.

Shoulder bone press: Sit up straight in a seat with your hands laying on your thighs. Hold your shoulders down and your jaw level. Gradually move your shoulders back and press your shoulder bones together. Hold for a count of five; unwind. Rehash three or multiple times.

Chest area stretch: Stand confronting a corner with your arms raised, hands level against the walls, elbows at shoulder level. Place one foot in front of the other. Bowing your forward knee, breathe out as you incline your body in the direction of the corner. Keep your back straight and your chest and head up. You ought to feel a pleasant stretch across your chest. Stand firm on this footing for 20-30 seconds. Unwind.

Arm-across-chest stretch: Raise your right arm to bear level before you and curve the arm at the elbow, keeping the lower arm lined up with the floor. Handle the right elbow with your left hand and delicately pull it across your chest so you feel a stretch in the upper arm and shoulder on the right side. Hold for 20 seconds; loosen up the two arms. Rehash to the opposite side. Rehash multiple times on each side.

Practice these symbolism and stance practices over the day. You could attempt to find a decent trigger to assist you with recollecting, for example, doing at least one of them when you get up from your work area, or just before booked breaks and lunch. Before long it will end up being a tendency.

16 Methods for staying away from Back Torment

If you've been sidelined by an irritating back, you're in good company. Four out of five individuals experience back torment eventually, making it the second most normal justification behind visiting the specialist.

Back torment takes different structures, from a tireless dull long to unexpected sharp torment, and has many causes. Some of the time it results from an injury, break, or other unplanned wounds. It can come from sickness or ailment, like joint pain, fibromyalgia, or spinal stenosis (a restricting of the spinal trench through which the spinal rope runs). Many individuals foster back torment to some degree since they're overweight or stationary.

Fortunately, lower back torment typically gets better within a couple of days or weeks, and medical procedure is seldom vital. Additionally, basic self-improvement systems, for example, can be shockingly successful at keeping back agony and holding it back from returning:

1. Get more activity: Assuming your back is harmed, you might figure the most ideal way to get help is to restrict exercise and rest. A little while of rest might help, yet more than that may not help the aggravation. Specialists presently

realize that ordinary actual work can assist with facilitating aggravation and muscle pressure.

Ask your health center instructor about back-reinforcing works out. Additionally, a few types of yoga and kendo may assist you with learning legitimate stances and further develop strength, equilibrium, and adaptability.

2. Watch your weight: Additional pounds, particularly in your midriff, can exacerbate back torment by moving your focal point of gravity and overwhelming your lower back. Remaining inside 10 pounds of your ideal weight might assist with controlling back torment.

3. Assuming you smoke, stop. Smoking limits the progression of supplements containing blood to spinal plates, so smokers are particularly helpless against back torment.

4. Rest soundly: If you're inclined to back torment, talk with your primary care physician about the best dozing position. Resting on your side with your knees pulled up somewhat toward your chest is at times proposed. Like to rest on your back? Set one pillow under your knees and one more under your lower back.

Dozing on your stomach can be particularly severe with your back. On the off odds that you can't rest differently, place a pillow under your hips.

Individuals lean toward various things on their sleeping pads. If it's too delicate, many individuals will have spinal pains. The equivalent is valid for extremely hard bedding. Numerous specialists suggest medium-supportive bedding for those with constant spinal pain. It might take experimentation to find what works for you. A piece of pressed wood between the container spring and sleeping cushion will solidify a delicate bed. A thick sleeping cushion will assist with mellowing excessively hard bedding.

5. Focus on your stance: First, really take a look at your stance by remaining with your heels against a wall. Your calves, rump, shoulders, and the rear of your head ought to contact the wall. You ought to have the option to slip your hand behind the little of your back. Presently, step forward and stand regularly. Assuming that your stance changes, right it immediately.

6. Begin with your seat: The best seat for forestalling back torment is unified with a straight back or low-back help. Keep your knees without a doubt higher than your hips while situated. Your seat back ought to be set at a point of around 110Try not to type on your telephone. Sending an incidental message or email on your phone is alright. Be that as it may, recollect, that when you type on your telephone, you're bowing your head and bending your spine. Assuming you do that for more than a couple of moments, it will place weight on the fragile vertebrae in your neck. The arrangement is basic. Save longer directives for when you can take a seat at a PC with a straight spine.

10. Enjoy a ton of reprieves: Like clockwork, require no less than 20 seconds to quit composing and stand and stretch. What's more, like clockwork, regardless of whether you enjoyed some time in the middle, stand and spend no less than 2 minutes from your PC. This gets your blood siphoning and relaxes tight muscles and solid joints. It likewise allows your eyes an opportunity to rearrange, which can forestall PC-related vision issues.

11. Watch out for how you lift: Don't twist around from the midsection to lift weighty articles. Twist your knees and squat, pulling in your stomach muscles and holding the item near your body as you stand up. Allow your legs to do the lifting, not your back. Try not to contort your body while lifting. If you would be able, push as opposed to pulling weighty items. Pushing is simpler on the back.

12. Keep away from high heels: They can move your focal point of gravity and strain your lower back. Adhere to a one-inch heel. If you need to go higher, bring along a couple of low-obeyed shoes and slip into them if you become awkward.

13. Stash the thin pants: Attire so close that it disrupts bowing, sitting, or strolling can bother back torment.

14. Ease up your wallet: Sitting on an overstuffed wallet might cause uneasiness and back torment. If you will be sitting for a drawn-out period - - while driving, for instance, removes your wallet from your back pocket.

15. Pick the right satchel or portfolio: Purchase a sack or folder case with a wide, customizable

lash that is sufficiently long to arrive at over your head. A courier pack (like the one bicycle couriers wear) is made to wear along these lines. Having the lash on the contrary shoulder of the pack disseminates the weight all the more equitably and assists keep your shoulders with night and your back aggravation free. While conveying a weighty sack or case without lashes, switch hands habitually to try not to put all the weight on one side of the body. To relieve the burden, occasionally cleanse packs, cases, knapsacks, and different transporters of things you needn't bother with.

16. Disregard back supports: Different back upholds are accessible, from flexible groups to unique bodices. They can be useful after specific sorts of medical procedures, yet there isn't a lot of proof that they assist with treating persistent back torment.

5 Stance Tips for an Aggravation Free Day

1. Standing: Keep your feet an agreeable distance separated, commonly something like the broadness of your shoulders with equivalent weight disseminated on every leg. Envision an upward line drawn from the focal point of your head through your shoulders and down to your pelvis. This is your ideal standing stance. On the off chance that your occupation expects you to represent delayed periods, consider utilizing a footstool to facilitate the strain. If you want extra back help, consistent yourself with a table or ledge, making sure to keep your head raised and spine straight. People remaining in a similar spot all day ought to utilize an elastic mat on the floor to further develop solace.

2. Strolling: Notice how individuals walk and you'll see that a large number of us incline forward, making weight on the back. Stroll without straining neck muscles, while keeping your pelvis straight and head level. With a great stance, your head ought to nearly feel weightless.

Keep away from level footed, "stepping," however rather land delicately on the impact point, moving load onto the wad of the foot lastly the toes. Use handbags, packs, and knapsacks intended to limit back strain.

3. Sitting: With so many of us sitting in a work area the entire day, it's normal to get drained and begin slumping without seeing it. That's what to counter, make the most of the seat's highlights with your bottom pushed to the rear of the seat. When your pelvis upholds your weight, you'll see the way a lot simpler it is to keep up with a great stance. Your knees ought to twist at a right point and be about a similar level as your hips. Utilize a little footstool under your feet to accomplish a legitimate position if necessary. Stay away from unequal stances like intersecting legs unevenly, inclining aside, slouching the shoulders, or shifting the head. Give your shoulders and back muscles a break by utilizing the armrests.

4. Lifting: Mistaken lifting can add to extreme, long-haul weakness. Given that, consistently plan before you lift. Keep protests your body instead of conveying with outstretched arms.

Indeed, even with light items, keep a straight back and use knee-bowing activities, not back-twisting activities. Fix your stomach muscles for additional help. Assuming lifting is essential for your normal day-to-day everyday practice, put resources into back help or other related hardware.

5. Working at the PC: as well as rehearsing a great sitting stance as recently examined, working at a PC expects you to keep your arms and wrists adjusted too. Pointless strain is put on the spine except if your seat, console, mouse, and PC screen are accurately situated.

Place your screen away from the glare and a good ways off of about a manageable distance when situated easily before it. Position the screen to your normal, resting eye position and try not to shift your head forward. Utilize a book or stand to raise it if necessary. Change your screen's brilliance, difference, and text dimension to agreeable levels. While composing, keep your arms lined up with your legs with great help under your wrists. Loosen up your upper arms and shoulders. If conceivable, place your reports straightforwardly before you.

Activities and tips for a better stance

The accompanying activities center around expanding muscle strength and adaptability for a better stance.

1. Spans

Spans assist with reinforcing the gluteal and muscular strength, which assuages the abundance of stress in the lower back.

To do an extension:

Lie on your back with your knees bowed and feet level on the floor.

Lift your hips by drawing in your center and bum muscles. The bum and lower back ought to raise off the ground.

Tenderly further down to the beginning position.

2. Board

Board Posture further develops pose by fortifying muscles in the shoulders and back as well as the center, glutes, and hamstrings. It likewise empowers the appropriate arrangement of the spine.

To board:

Get down onto your hands and knees. Ensure that your hands line up with your shoulders and your knees line up with your hips.

Go onto the chunks of the feet by lifting your impact points and fixing your legs. The body ought to shape a straight line.

Keep your chest open and shoulders back.

Stand firm on this footing for 30-60 seconds.

3. Hip flexor stretch

This stretch tenderly opens the hips and further develops equilibrium and coordination, which can assist with further developing stance.

To do a hip flexor stretch:

Bow with your right knee on the ground.

Place your left foot in front and twist your knee at a 90-degree point.

Keep your back straight, chest forward, and head upstanding.

Put two hands on your left thigh.

Delicately press your hips forward and stand firm on the footing for 20--30 seconds.

Rehash this stretch on the right side.

4. Mountain Posture

Tadasana, or Mountain Posture, is a straightforward yoga position that can assist with further developing stance. Mountain Posture centers around upstanding body arrangement, and it integrates a few parts of a good stance.

Stand upstanding with the feet hip-width separated.

Make a point to spread your weight equitably through the two feet. Attempt delicately shaking forward and in reverse to feel what varieties in weight dissemination mean for the pose.

Keep a slight twist in your knees, crush your thighs, and slant your tailbone down.

Drop your shoulders down and back, so your chest approaches

Keep your shoulders loose and permit your arms to tumble to the sides of the body with your palms looking ahead. Breathe in and breathe out leisurely for a couple of breaths.

5. Youngster's Posture

This yoga present protracts the lower back and opens the hips. Individuals can involve Youngster's Posture as a resting position during yoga or different types of activity or as a component of their standard extending schedule.

To do Kid's Posture:

Get down onto your hands and knees.

Tenderly lean your body in reverse, keeping your hands similarly situated.

Keep reclining until your brow contacts the floor.

Your arms ought to make a straight line and your bottom ought to lay behind you.

Keep your arms straight and shoulders loose.

Putting a mat or towel on the floor can make this posture more agreeable.

General ways to further develop pose:

Know about acting during ordinary exercises, like strolling, sitting in front of the TV, and finishing tasks.

Remain dynamic by participating in normal activity, including cardio, strength preparing, or extending.

Keep a sound weight, as additional weight can debilitate the abs and put weight on the joints and tendons.

Wear agreeable, low-obeyed shoes that have curve support. High-obeyed shoes modify an individual's focal point of gravity, which can put more weight on the muscles and joints, particularly in the knees.

Position work areas and tables at the right level of involving them in working or eating.

General tips for a good stance include:

Holding your shoulders back and chest forward holding your head upstanding, following your spine abstaining from bending at the midsection keeping the body's weight disseminated equally among the two feet and hips

Having a great stance can work on fearlessness and may give a few medical advantages, for example, diminished back torment, diminished chance of injury, lower weight on the muscles and joints.

Spinal pain and discomfort in pregnancy

Numerous ladies experience back torment while pregnant. Brought about by various elements influence your stance during pregnancy. You can change and support your stance to assist with working on low back torment.

Step-by-step instructions to diminish back torment during pregnancy

You can forestall back torment or decrease it by:

Wearing agreeable, steady, low-obeyed shoes, not representing extensive stretches.

Sitting with your base against the rear of a seat and sitting up tall - put a little pad on your lower back if necessary fold your hands under your knock for help on the off potential for success that having for significant stretches, not lifting weighty items - assuming you want to lift anything, twist your knees and hold a straight back, remaining dynamic with delicate activities and extending reinforcing your pelvic floor monitoring your stance

Right stance during pregnancy

The accompanying activity will assist with reinforcing the stomach (stomach) muscles that can support and move back torment during pregnancy.

Down on the ground, ensure your knees are under your hips and your hands are under your shoulders. Your spine ought to be straight and in a nonpartisan 'box' position.

1. Delicate turn

Sitting tall on your mat, legs crossed, feel both bum cheeks interface with the mat.

Tenderly bend/pivot to one side. This ought to feel good consistently, your bum cheeks remaining associated with the mat.

Keep breathing serenely.

Hold for 20 seconds.

Rehash multiple times.

Presently rehash this exercise yet turn to the right this time.

2. Hip Flexor Strech

Sit leg over leg on the mat.

Put your left hand on the floor as you delicately point your right arm up towards the roof.

Presently tenderly incline towards the left side. Both bum cheeks ought to keep in touch with the floor.

Take long, full breaths in this stance, permitting you tenderly unwind into this stretch.

Hold for 20 seconds.

Rehash multiple times.

Presently trade sides and play out a similar activity yet extending to one side.

3. Shellfish work out

This exercise ought to feel great and agony allowed to perform.

Lie on your left side with your back level against the wall. Twist your knees and spot your feet level against the wall.

Presently open and close your right knee.

Rehash multiple times or until your bum muscle starts to feel excessively drained to lift the knee.

Rest for 30 seconds.

Rehash 2 additional sets.

Presently change positions and rehash the activity lying on your right side.

4. Youngster's posture.

Stoop on the floor, with your knees spread wide and your feet near one another. This permits space for your child to knock.

Presently permit your bum to sit right back onto your heels. Place a pad at your heels if it feels better.

This ought to feel like an unwinding, agreeable stretch in your low back.

Reasons for back torment during pregnancy

Back torment is brought about by changes happening to your body to oblige your developing child: your muscles and connective tissues stretch as your child develops, your stance changes to oblige the expanded weight you're conveying, and changing chemicals can cause your pelvis and back to feel more vulnerable there's additional pressure and less help for the joints in your back.

How not to help great sitting stance

That is not all. While there are a lot of tips to sit well, remember these "don'ts" of sitting stance:

Try not to incline forward toward your PC. That comes down on your lower back.

Try not to incline in reverse. That can make you droop, overwhelming your back. To figure out the perfect balance between excessively far forward or in reverse, rock this way and that and afterward land in the center and remain there.

Try not to overarch your back. Try not to curve at the midriff in your turning office seat. Turn your entire body. Remember to slide to the front of your seat before you stand up.

Try not to sit for over 30 minutes. Get up, move around, stretch, and relax!

Try not to droop. If you end up sinking into a rut, utilize a lumbar roll between your lower back and the seat for help. Remember to relax. Great tummy breathing can assist you with keeping away from a throbbing pain.

www.ingramcontent.com/pod-product-compliance
Lightning Source LLC
LaVergne TN
LVHW020536160826
845677LV00015B/4100
9798845835543